ACUPRESSURE

By
Nancy Shiffrin
And
Sharon Lee Bailey

MAJOR BOOKS • CANOGA PARK, CALIFORNIA

MB

CONTENTS

INTRODUCTION

I have been practicing acupressure in the Los Angeles area for a number of years. In that time I have also given workshops at Esalen, Big Sur, Asilomar, Monterey, and Topanga Center.

I have had occasion to see the great value of acupressure. I have seen people learn to relax themselves, treat their own minor health problems, and work with partners to increase and maintain sexual pleasure.

Acupressure as a treatment is being validated now by the many acupuncture research projects in Los Angeles. At UCLA, research is being done on the value of acupuncture for treatment of pain and for obesity.

At the University of Southern California-Los Angeles County Hospital, acupuncture research is being done to explain and define acupuncture in terms of Western medicine. In fact, using heat photography, they are showing that the meridians, discussed in detail in this book, follow the major pathways of the nerves.

Dr. Gerald Looney, head of the USC-Los Angeles County project told me he uses acupressure, or finger pressure, as he prefers to call it, on himself and teaches it to his friends. "You can't go wrong with do-it-yourself acupressure," Dr. Looney says.

My own experience has borne this out. If you follow the instructions in this book, and pay attention to the warnings I have provided, your health, beauty, and vitality will be at your fingertips.

Sharon Bailey

Chapter One

WHAT IS ACUPRESSURE?

Acupressure is a form of massage that makes use of the acupuncture pressure points. Instead of a doctor using needles on your pressure points, he uses the pressure of his fingers. You can learn to do it yourself, or with a partner. And you can control your health and your appearance; your pleasure is literally at your fingertips!

Acupressure is sometimes known as *shiatsu*. This is a Japanese word meaning *shi* (fingers) and *atsu* (pressure).The Japanese use finger pressure to treat and prevent illness, and to maintain optimum physical conditioning.

But it is not merely a remedy. Acupressure affects your total outlook on life, stimulating your own body's power to prevent illness and maintain health.

Jin Shin Jyutsu is another form of acupressure, this based on the healing power of touch.

How Did Acupressure Begin?

Some experts say that the history of acupressure begins with the story of acupuncture. Others feel it is as basic as the first man holding his foot because it hurt, or touching his mate because she wasn't feeling well.

Somewhere in the early history of man, experts theorize, people began to discover that touching was not only pleasant, it was therapeutic. They began to notice that touching a particular part of the body caused pain to be relieved in other parts of the body.

Soon man began to establish a relationship between certain points on the body and the flow of some kind of energy between these points. By tuning into that energy flow, he was even able to map it out in detailed anatomical patterns. Today, modern scientific research is verifying the accuracy of these patterns.

Dr. Gerald Looney, of the USC Medical School, reports taking pictures of the energy flow along nerve pathways by way of thermography (heat photography). These nerve pathways match the meridians, or lines of energy flow, that the Orientals mapped thousands of years ago.

Man discovered that needles could conduct this energy that flowed through human fingertips. This made it easier for doctors and healers to give treatments, because it neither drained the doctor of his own energy, nor forced him to absorb the patient's stagnated energy.

Professional Oriental therapists and doctors thus turned extensively to the use of needles, while the primitive finger-pressure method remained largely a folk therapy.

Today, however, there is a great revival of Oriental folk therapies, or natural healing arts. Yoga, *T'ai Ch'i,* macrobiotics, herbal remedies, have all gained in popularity in the United States in the past decade.

Certain Oriental techniques, such as aikido, acupuncture, and karate, demand a master's participation. Others, such as acupressure, are available to some extent to the laymen.

What Is the Theory Behind Acupressure?

Oriental medicine is based on a total concept of the whole person. Western medicine is based on a physical cure of a symptom. For example, if you have ulcers and go to a Western doctor, he will probably give you medicine for the ulcers and prescribe a special diet.

Asked to treat the same difficulty, the Oriental doctor will discuss your life-style, your eating, sleeping and drinking habits, as they relate to your problem. He might even ask you to discuss your philosophy of life.

In conjunction with treating your ulcer, he will consider you, the total person, and your way of life.

I must add a word of caution here. If you have any persisting symptom, any serious disease, even the hint of a thought that you might, visit a doctor. Acupressure is not a substitute for medical care. It is an adjunct, and it is extremely valuable in the treatment of minor health problems, beauty problems related to skin care, and it is valuable in assisting you and your partner in obtaining more joy and pleasure out of sex.

Acupressure, and its sister art, acupuncture, work through the energy that flows in the body, along imaginary lines called meridians.

These paths end at various points in the body, which we will refer to as pressure points. Western researchers are verifying that the *chi*, or energy, that Oriental literature describes, is in fact, nerve impulses you stimulate by pressing the points.

Can I Really Learn to Do It Myself?

Yes. You will learn to trust your body's natural power to heal itself. Acupressure is as natural as breathing. It is as natural as two people touching to show they care.

When your neck is tense, you rub it. When your child is sick, you massage his chest. When your partner is tired, you give him, or her, a back rub.

Acupressure is as simple and natural as this, only more sophisticated. If you make a mistake, there will be no benefit, but you won't do any harm, either.

Although complicated illnesses and chronic conditions require the attention of specialists, you can treat yourself for simple difficulties, by using the easy-to-follow acupressure techniques described in this book.

Can I Really Learn to Apply Acupressure With a Partner?

Yes. There are a few simple rules:
1. Do not treat anyone for a serious disease.
2. If a symptom, such as a headache, persists or reoccurs, see a doctor.

3. Never press to the point of pain. Leave complicated treatments to a master.

When Should I Consult a Master?

For certain illnesses, for anaesthesia, or to learn more advanced techniques, consultation with a master, an expert in applying acupressure, is advised. The treatments in this book are designed to help you achieve greater health, improved appearance, greater relaxation and greater pleasure in life, particularly in your sex life!

Since certain serious health conditions do respond to acupressure, many acupressure masters work hand in hand with medical doctors, in the treatment of a variety of problems.

Chapter Two

HOW TO DO IT

Correct Use of the Hands

It is your thumbs that you will most frequently use when applying acupressure treatments, either to yourself or to a partner. Usually you will press down with the bulb of your thumb. Seldom will you press forward with the tip, since this can tire or even injure your hand.

When you treat your face and abdomen, however, the index, middle and ring fingers, will come into play.

Needless to say, your fingernails should be trimmed short to avoid hurting yourself or your partner.

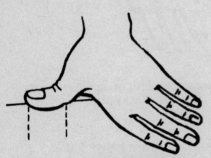

a. Correct   b. Wrong   c. Wrong

Pressure is applied with the ball of the thumb.

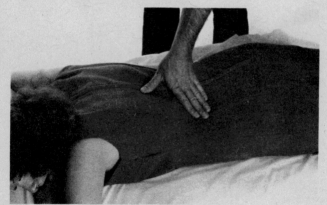

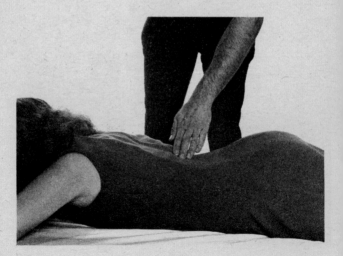

Here, finger pressure is applied, using three fingers. Sometimes, the ball of thumb may also be used.

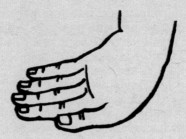

In this case, the palm is used.

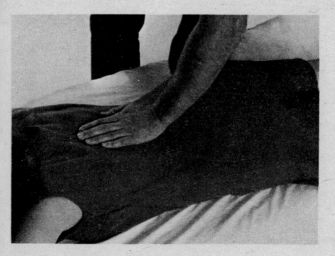

How to Apply Pressure

Never jab your fingers into your partner's flesh. Apply firm pressure with the soft bulbs of your fingers, as if you were resting all your body weight on them. The degree of pressure required depends on the symptoms and the person's condition. Your posture, however, should be such that, if it becomes necessary, you can apply your entire weight. The area of contact between the thumb and the body of the partner should be about the same as that inked on paper when fingerprints are taken. Pressure should be gentle, never to the point of pain, and perpendicular to the area being treated.

Which Pressure Points to Treat

When you go to a master, he will treat all points on the body, before he treats you for a specific complaint. In do-it-yourself acupressure, it is wise to limit treatments to the specific points. The treatments I will describe will last about three minutes each.

There is one exception to this. If you are fatigued or tense, or your partner is, it is best to treat this problem before you attempt to treat anything else.

Usually you will treat points nearest the sight of the complaint. That is, to treat headaches, you will treat the muscles in the neck and scalp. There will be times, however, that the treatments recommended for a specific problem will involve points that are distant from the affected area.

This, because the energy flowing to one part of the body may be controlled by an organ in a distant part of the body. For example, the stomach meridian controls skin appearance.

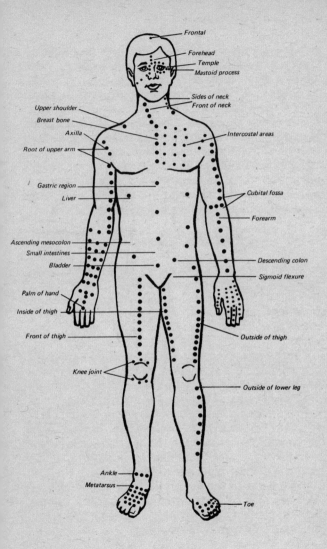

19

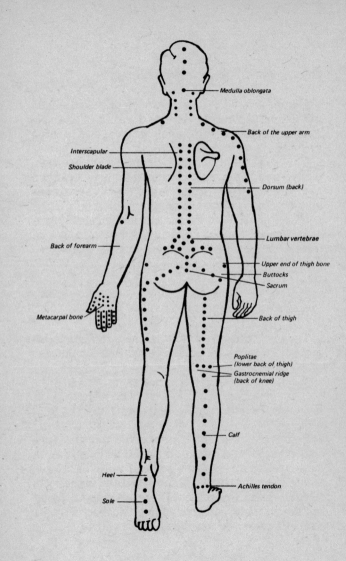

Medulla oblongata

Back of the upper arm

Interscapular

Shoulder blade

Dorsum (back)

Lumbar vertebrae

Back of forearm

Upper end of thigh bone

Buttocks

Sacrum

Metacarpal bone

Back of thigh

Poplitae
(lower back of thigh)

Gastrocnemial ridge
(back of knee)

Calf

Heel

Achilles tendon

Sole

Duration and Degree of Pressure

Except around the neck, where pressure should not exceed three seconds, the duration of a single application of pressure should be from five to seven seconds.

The sensation should be midway between pleasure and pain. A professional acupressurist can apply pressure that produces deep bodily sensations and benefit—without causing any discomfort.

Under clinical conditions, normally healthy persons usually undergo about thirty minutes of treatment, and invalids, about one hour. You are asked not to treat anyone for more than a few minutes at a time.

Position During Treatment

The ideal position during an acupressure treatment permits total rest and relaxation for the person treated.

With acupuncture, it is necessary to have the patient in a reclining position. The advantage of acupressure, however, is that you can do it anywhere.

People have given themselves acupressure treatments while riding on a bus, while sitting in first-class on an airplane, while at work, as fatigue and tension build up, at home in bed and in the bath, to name just a few places. There are many types of applications you can give yourself so discreetly, no one will know you are doing it.

Chapter Three

ACUPRESSURE FOR YOUR GOOD HEALTH

What does it mean to be healthy? You know you're healthy when you wake up each morning ready to deal with life, when you don't really want to stay in bed, when you are not plagued by minor ailments.

What has acupressure to do with your health? If you've had a problem with diarrhea, constipation, hangovers, stiff neck, headaches, migraine, colds, blood pressure, whiplash, sore or swollen throat, back pain, hemorrhoids, foot care, asthma and related allergies, and other minor health problems, acupressure may be your answer—your cure!

Of course, I cannot stress enough that it is wise to see a doctor before engaging in any do-it-yourself treatments to guarantee you do not have a severe condition requiring medical attention. For example, headaches might be symptomatic of tumors. In this case, you are obviously not qualified to treat a tumor.

Acupressure is most valuable when used to maintain your health and free yourself from the minor physical difficulties that interfere with your daily functioning.

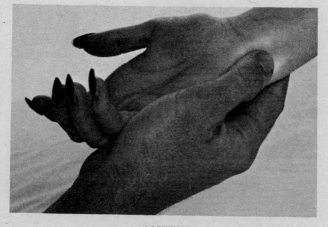

ANXIETY

Along the side of the wrist near the little finger, in the joint between wrist and hand, there is a tender spot.

In a lying down or sitting position, use your thumbnail to press hard.

ARM ACHE

Bend your elbow to a 90-degree angle. Locate the point at the outside end of the crease. In a lying down or sitting position, use your thumb to press hard.

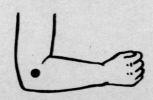

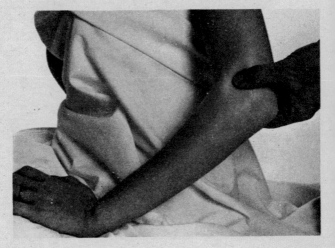

ASTHMA

Locate the point at the base of the neck. If you feel around the bony rim of your neck, you will find a slight depression in the center.

In a sitting or lying down position, use your index finger to press inward and downward.

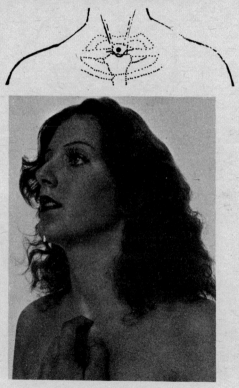

Locate the point between the shoulder blades, about one and one-half inches to the side of the third thoracic disk. This will be a tender spot about two inches above the mid-line of the shoulder blade.

Place partner in a sitting or lying down position, and use your thumbs to massage hard toward the disk.

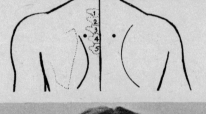

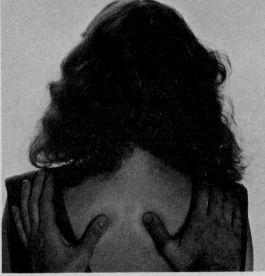

Find the points three inches to the side of the lower end of the fourth thoracic disk.

This technique again calls for a partner. While you are in a sitting position, or lying down on your stomach, have your partner use his thumbs to massage hard.

BEDWETTING

The points for treatment of bedwetting lie in the little finger, at the center of the creases of the top two knuckles.

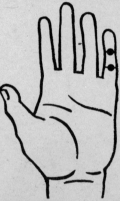

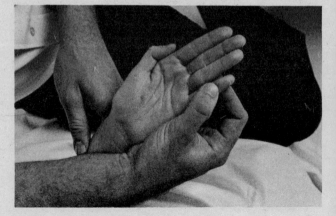

You should be sitting down or lying down when you do this treatment. Use your thumbnail to press hard on point number one. If you do not get results, use both points, first treating number one, then number two.

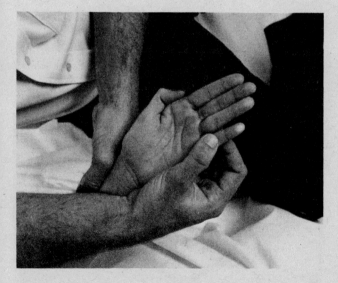

CONSTIPATION

Find the point four inches below the navel, just at the top of the groin area, at the midpoint of the abdominal area.

In a lying down position, use the thumb to press hard.

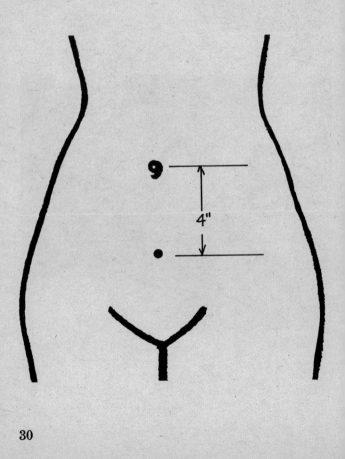

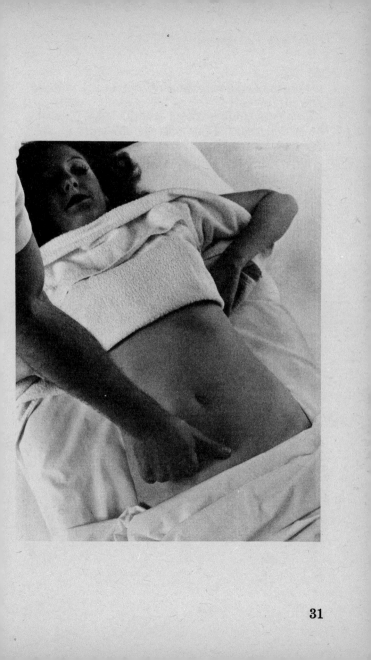

Locate the point between the tip of the tailbone and the anus.

In a lying down position, use the index finger to press downward. Then massage upward.

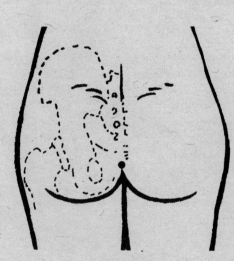

DIZZINESS

Locate the tender spot in between your eyebrows. Either sitting or lying down, use your thumb and index finger to pinch hard.

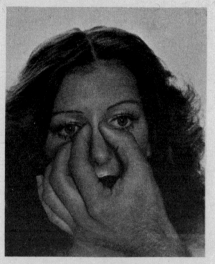

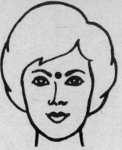

This treatment involves the foot. There is a point about two inches from the juncture of the big toe and first toe, in the depression between the first and second metatarsal bones.

You should be in a sitting or lying down position to treat this point. Press hard with the thumbnail.

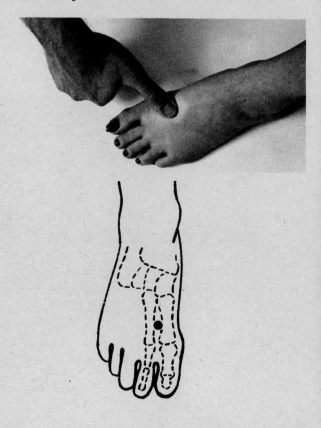

EXCESSIVE PERSPIRATION

You can control excessive sweating with this technique. Locate the point at the center of the palm.

Lie or sit down. Press hard with your thumbnail.

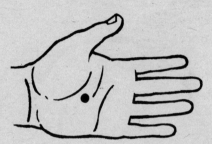

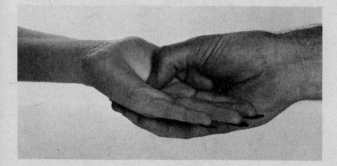

FAINTING

There is a point midway between your nose and the top of your lips. In a lying down or sitting position, press hard with either thumb or your index finger.

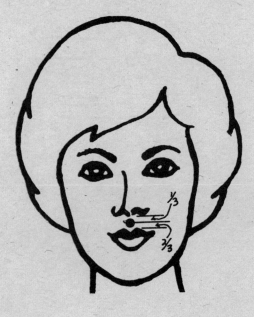

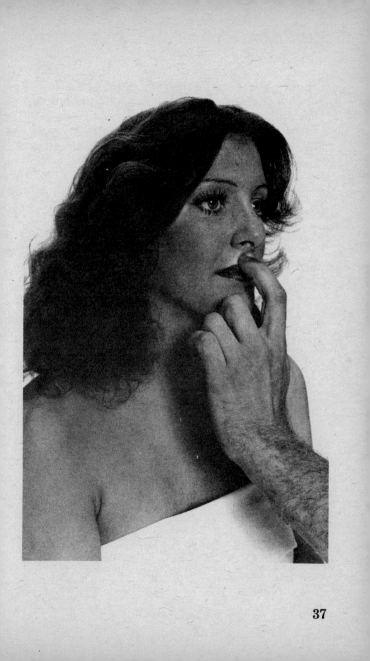

Locate the point at the front third of the foot, between the second and third metatarsal bones, beneath the calloused pads.

Treat your partner in a lying-down position. Using your thumbnail, press hard on this point.

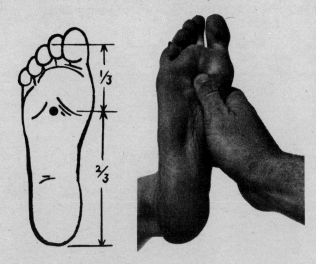

HEADACHES

There is a tender spot on the back of the hand, between the thumb and first finger. Specifically, it is located between the first and second metacarpal bones.

In a lying down or seated position, use your thumb to press against the second metacarpal bone, the one extending from the bone of your index finger.

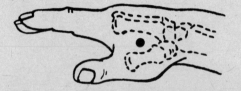

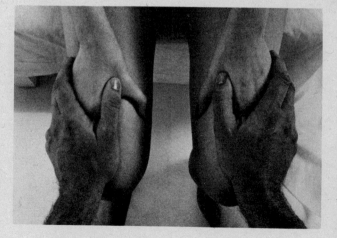

Locate the points below the bones of the skull on either side of the back of the neck, and about one and one-half inches to either side of the midline of the head.

Sit down and bend the head forward. Use your thumb to massage hard, treating both points simultaneously.

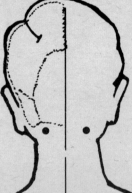

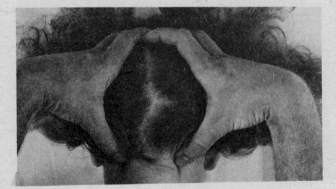

HEAT STROKE

Find the point between the nose and the top of the lips. In a lying down or sitting position, press hard with your thumb or your index finger.

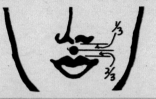

At the front one-third of the sole of the foot, between the second and third metatarsal bones, press hard using your thumbnail.

You should be lying down for this one.

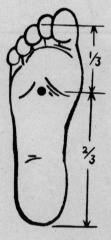
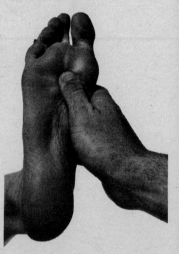

HYSTERIA

At the center of the bottom crease of the thumb, press hard with the thumbnail. Any posture is acceptable for this treatment.

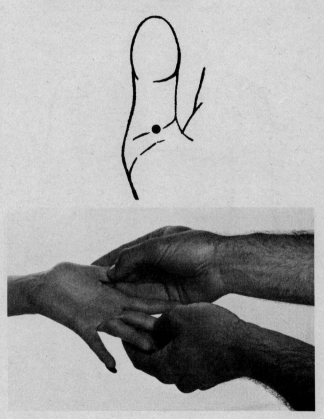

INTESTINAL STRESS

Locate the point four inches above the navel, along the center of the abdomen.

In a sitting or reclining position, use the thumb or palm of the hand to massage inward.

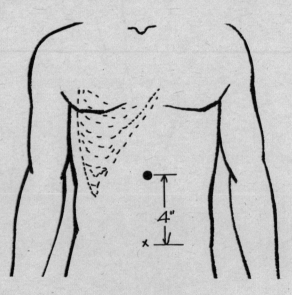

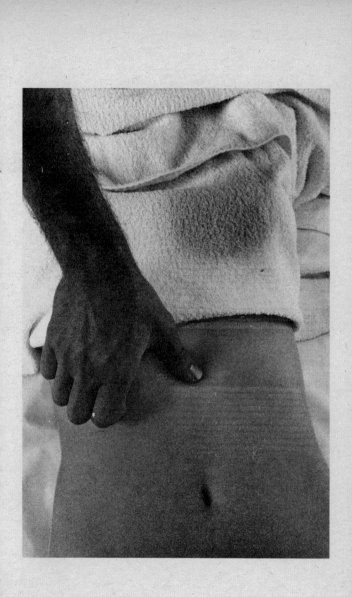

Locate the point three inches below the kneecap, one inch to the outside of the bone which runs up the front of the leg.

In a seated or reclining position, use the thumb to press down, then massage gently upward.

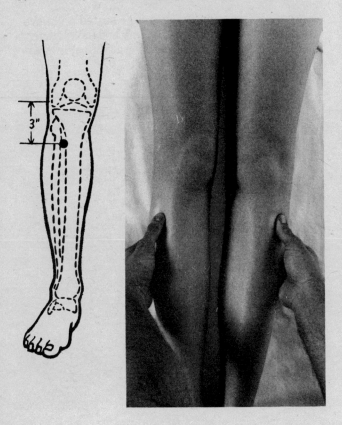

KNEE PAIN

There are pressure points in the depressions below the kneecap on either side of the bone. You can find them by pressing the area until you reach the tender spot.

For this treatment you must be seated and have your knee bent. Using your thumb and index finger, press hard on the two depressions at the same time.

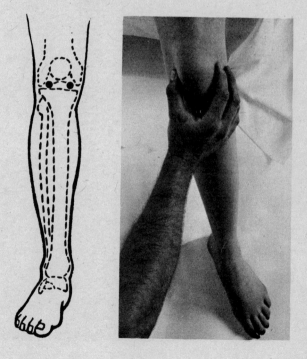

LOWER BACK PAIN

There are pressure points all along your spine. To treat pain in the lower back, locate the points one and one-half inches to each side of the second lumbar disk.

Lying down on your stomach, have your partner press hard with his thumbs toward the center of your spine.

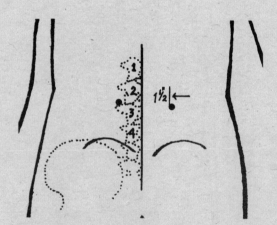

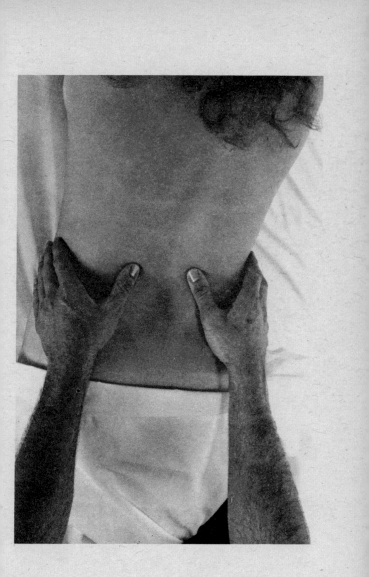

Locate the point on the large muscle of the shoulder, on a line with the nipple.

In a sitting position, have your partner use his thumbs over the point, and his fingers over the rest of the muscle.

Squeeze and release. Repeat this treatment for about sixty seconds.

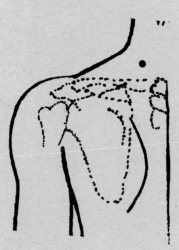

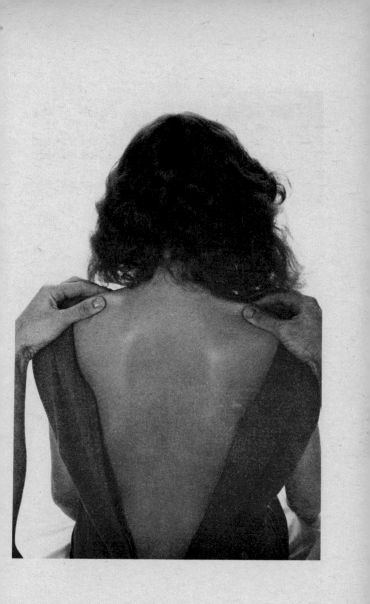

Locate the points below the bone of the skull. These are about one and one-half inches to either side of the midline of the head.

Use your thumbs to massage hard.

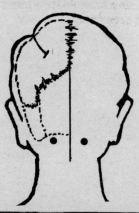

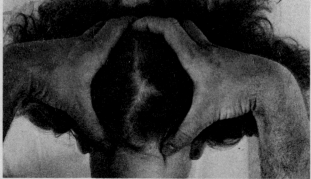

PALPITATION

Locate the point on the inside of the wrist, along-side the tendon that runs up the side of the arm.
In a lying down or sitting position, use your thumbnail to press hard.

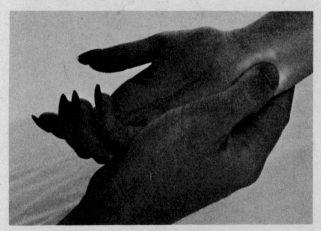

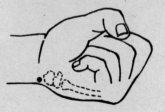

SHORTNESS OF BREATH

Locate the tender spot in the center of the neckbone. There is an indentation in the center of the bone. For this treatment you should be lying or sitting down.

Using your index finger, press inward, then massage down.

At the base of the neck, on either side of the spinal column, are two points. Have your partner sit down and bend his head forward.

Using your thumbs, massage hard toward the center of the spine.

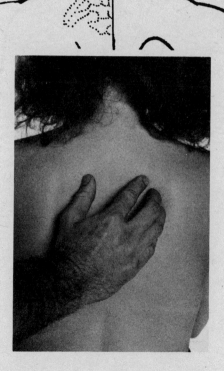

About one and one-half inches to the side of the top of the shoulder blade, there are tender spots.

For this treatment you should be sitting down or lying on your stomach. Have your partner massage hard toward the center of the spine.

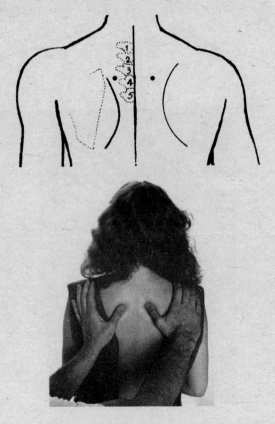

Measuring with your thumb knuckles, go about four inches from the base of the neck down your partner's spine. Find the points three inches to either side of the spine.

For this treatment, have your partner sit or lie down on his stomach. Use your thumbs to massage hard.

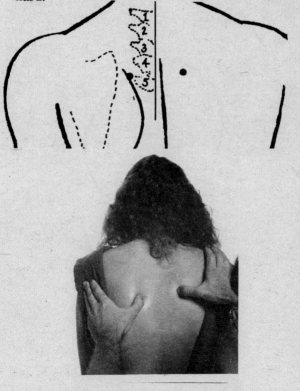

SHOULDER ACHE

At the front of the shoulder, just below the bone, there is a tender spot.

In a sitting position, use your thumb to press hard.

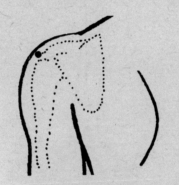

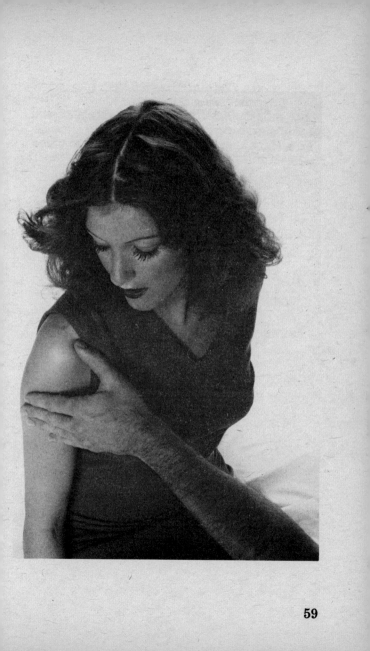

On the shoulder muscle, along the same line as the nipple, there is a pressure point.

Use your thumbs over your partner's points, and your fingers over his shoulder. While he is in a sitting position, squeeze hard and release.

Repeat this procedure for about one minute.

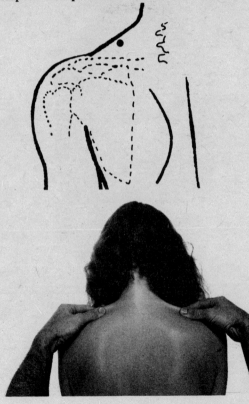

SINUS

Locate the point midway between the eyebrows. In a lying down or sitting position, use your thumbs to press hard.

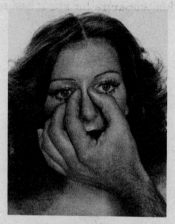

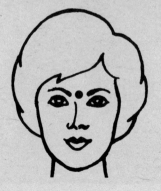

There are two tender spots at the side of the nose, just outside the nostrils. In a lying down or sitting position, use your index fingers to massage this point.

SLEEPLESSNESS

There is a point at the base of the calf muscle, about three inches above the middle of the ankle.
In a lying down or sitting position, use your thumb to press hard.

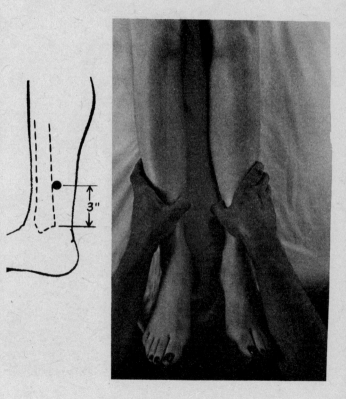

There is a point about one inch behind and slightly above the lobe of the ear near the rim of the skull.

In lying down or sitting position, use your index finger to press hard.

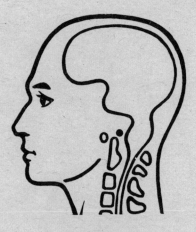

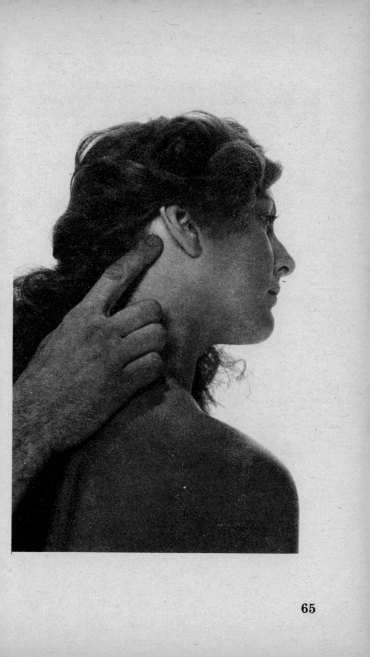

On the inside of the wrist, palm facing you, locate the point in the joint, where wrist and hand join.

In a lying down or sitting position, use your thumbnail to press hard.

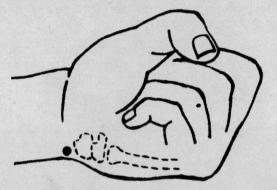

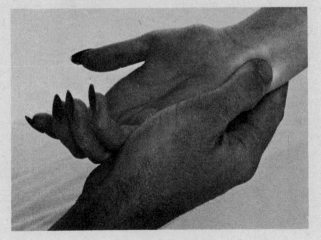

SORE THROAT

Locate the point one-half inch away from the corner of your thumbnail.

The posture is not important for this one. Use your thumbnail to press hard.

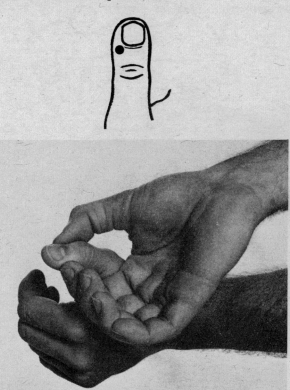

Over the back of the hand, between the bones of the thumb and first finger, there is a tender spot. You can tell you have found the spot when you find the groove or indentation in the bone.

Sitting, lying down or standing, use your thumbs to press hard against the second bone, the one which extends from the index finger.

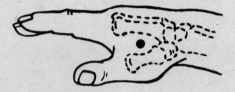

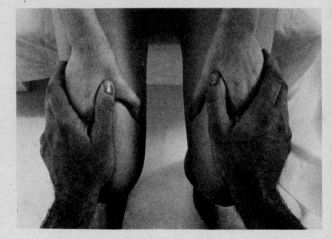

At the front one-third of the sole of the foot, just below and to the inside of the large callous, there is an important pressure point.

This treatment is most efficient if you lie down. Have your partner use his thumbnail to press hard.

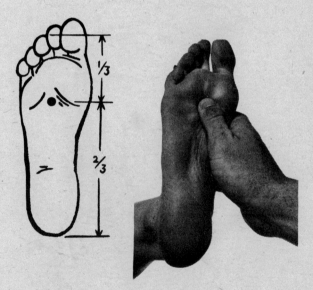

TENSION IN THE JAW

Over the jaw muscle, in the angle of the jawbone, there is a tender spot.

In a sitting or lying down position, using both thumbs, massage both points at the same time.

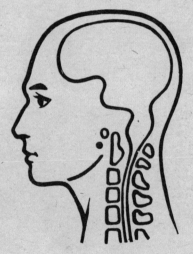

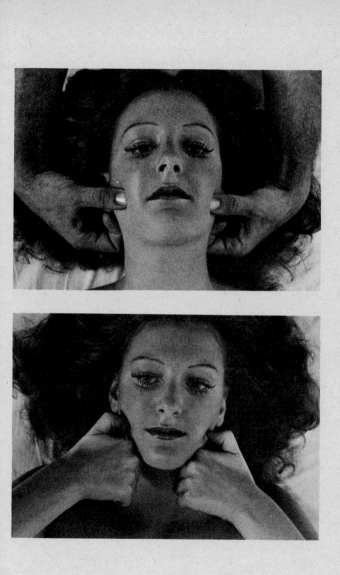

71

TOOTHACHE

This treatment is good for upper jaw, lower jaw or both.

Over the back of the hand, between the thumb and first finger, there is a groove between the bones.

Locate the tender spot in that groove. Lie or sit down. Use your thumb to press against the bone extending from the index finger.

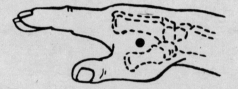

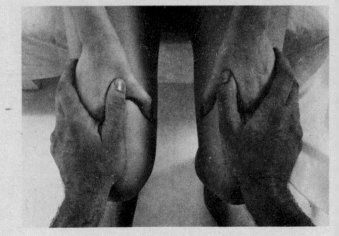

There is a tender point about one inch in front of the opening of the ear.

In a lying down position, use your thumbs to press hard.

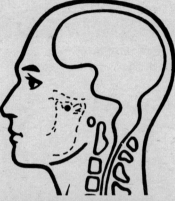

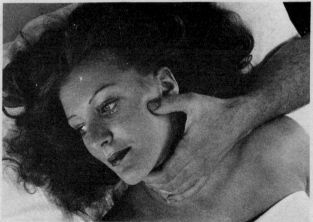

There is a point at the bend in the large bone of the jaw.

In a sitting down or lying down position, use your thumbs to massage hard.

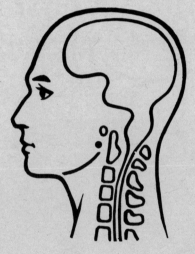

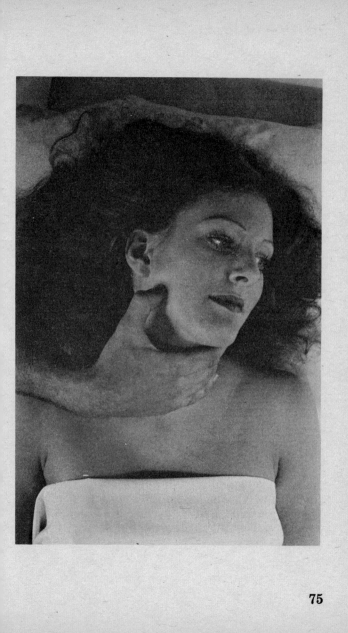

Chapter Four

HEIGHTEN YOUR SEXUAL PLEASURE

In this chapter, you will learn some of the long-buried secrets of the Orient. And like countless of other happy couples, you can discover how to use acupressure to improve your sex life.

Using the following techniques, many women have become more responsive, have improved the frequency and strength of their orgasms, increased their vitality and attractiveness.

Men may benefit from do-it-yourself acupressure in a number of ways. Those suffering from premature ejaculation may find relief and learn control. Men who are losing potency may regain it. And many men report an increasing sense of youthfulness and vitality as a result of do-it-yourself acupressure.

One of the secrets of the Orient is that partners are not bashful about communicating what they want in the bedroom. Many of these procedures can be done with a partner. Because you are working so closely and intimately with your partner, it is possible your communication will improve enormously. Many couples who practice acupressure report these benefits.

IMPOTENCE

Have your partner locate the pressure point three inches below your kneecap, and one inch to the outside of your shinbone.

While you are in a lying down position, have her use her thumb to press down, then massage upward.

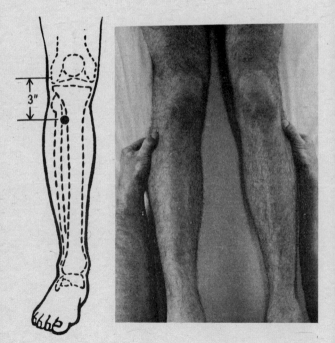

About one and one-half inches to the side of the lower end of the second lumbar disk, there are two points, one on each side of the spinal column.

In a sitting down or lying down position, have your partner use her thumbs to press hard toward the spine.

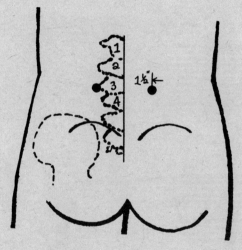

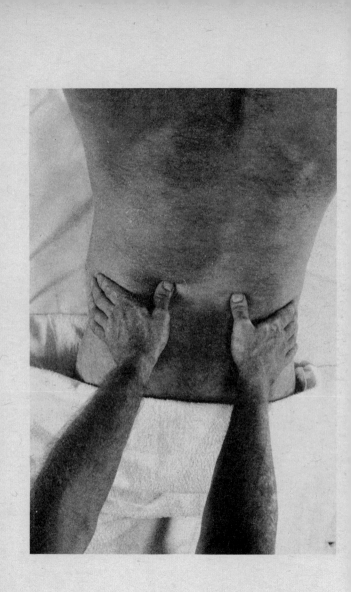

Locate the point three inches below the navel, along the midline of the abdomen.

Lying down, use your thumb or palm to massage hard.

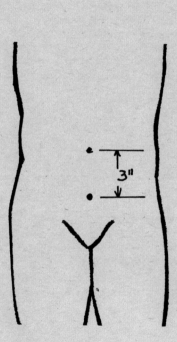

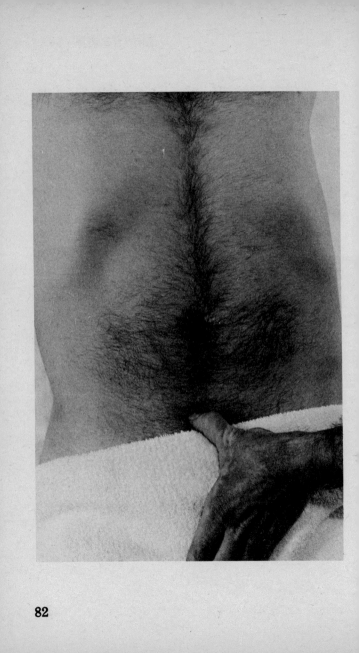

Locate the point about three inches above the middle of the ankle, behind your shinbone.

While you are in a reclining position, have your partner use her thumbs to press hard.

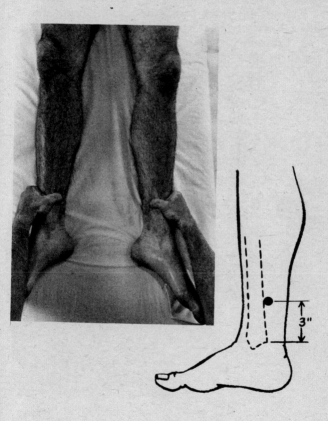

CONTROL OF EJACULATION

Here's a treatment for young men who have difficulty controlling ejaculation. It should also help the more experienced, older man in performing several times a night, with only one ejaculation.

1. Press the three points along the sacrum, the lower back area, for three to seven seconds.

2. Press the point right between the breastbone, for three to seven seconds.

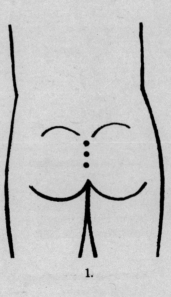

1.

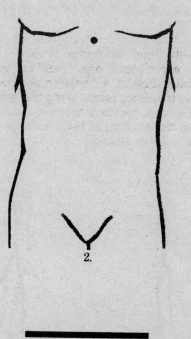

2.

Another way to control premature ejaculation: Locate the sensitive point at the tip of the penis. Using the thumb and index finger, squeeze the tip of the penis while the penis is still erect, just before orgasm.

THE LIVER

Poorly functioning livers, common among people in sedentary occupations, decrease sexual potency. To treat the liver, locate the point beneath the right rib, and apply pressure frequently.

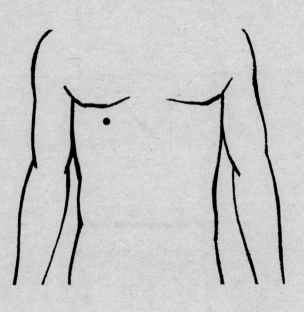

BOWELS

Constipation weakens the flow of energy through the body, thereby weakening sex.

To stimulate bowel movement, locate the spot left of the navel, just above and to the right of the juncture between the left leg and hip.

Knead this area gently.

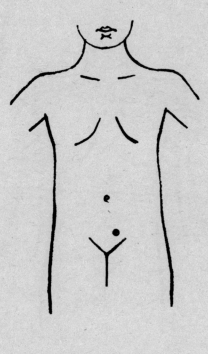

THE BLADDER

Stimulation of the bladder increases sexual response.

Locate the point in the groin area, at the border of the pubic hair.

When the male massages this area gently, it will increase sensitivity in his testicles.

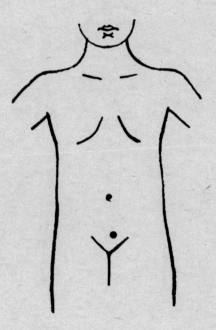

IMPROVE FEMALE SEXUAL RESPONSE

Locate the point that affects the thyroid gland. Do this by pressing the point in front of the neck, above the collarbone or clavicle. Press for five to seven seconds.

This pressure on the endocrine glands will stimulate sexual sensitivity in the woman.

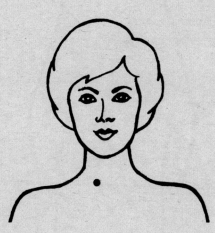

With a partner, locate the points above the suprarenal glands, located in the small of your back.

Lying on your stomach, have your partner apply pressure to these glands with his fist.

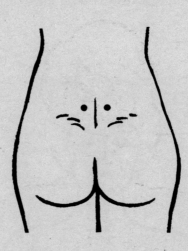

Locate the points between your breasts. There is an endocrine gland behind the breasts, and the points governing it are in two rows between the breasts. There are four on each side.

Apply pressure with your fingers for from five to seven seconds.

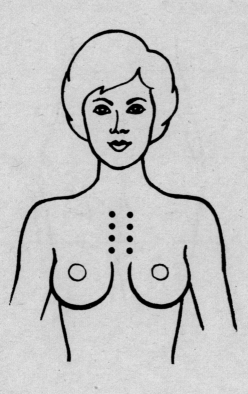

THE THIGHS

Locate, or have your partner locate, the points on the thighs, at the juncture between the hip and leg, inside the joint.

Apply pressure, or have your partner apply pressure, for five to seven seconds.

Treating this area heightens a woman's sexual response.

PREVENTING LOSS OF SEXUAL ENERGY

Locate the points above the sacrum. This is the area in the lowermost part of your back.

Lying on your stomach, have your partner apply pressure for five to seven seconds on each point.

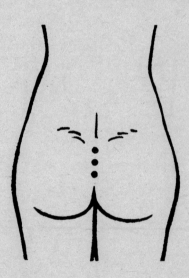

TREATING FRIGIDITY

1. Have the woman rest on her stomach.
2. Working downward, with all the weight of your body, press both sides of the third, fourth and fifth lumbar vertebrae.
3. Next, gently, press the points on the buttocks.

Lumbar vertebrae

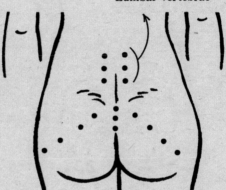

MENOPAUSE

Menopause is a natural life process. It's symptoms, however, are often uncomfortable. For relief of such symptoms as dizziness, sweating, loss of appetite, moodiness, excitability, chronic headache, etc., try the following acupressure treatment:

Locate the points on the throat which control the thyroid gland. With the thumb and four fingers, apply pressure for about thirty seconds. Detailed treatment of ongoing discomfort should involve the assistance of a master.

Chapter Five

A BREAST BEAUTIFICATION PROGRAM

You can enlarge, firm and shape your breasts using acupressure. Here are some suggested treatments, which have proven effective with hundreds of women.

1. Locate the points on your neck that control your thyroid gland. They are on both sides of the long cord. Using your thumb and three fingers, massage for from three to five seconds.

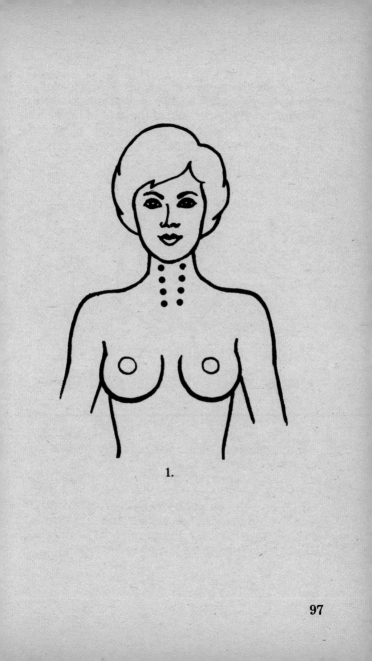

1.

2. Locate the point which controls the medulla oblongata or lower brain. It is located at the base of the skull, at the upper part of the back of the neck. Have partner press his thumbs on this point for from five to seven seconds.

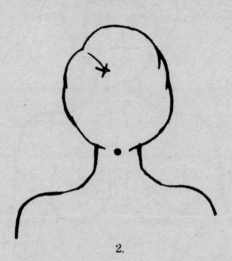

2.

3. Locate the points on the upper shoulder. Have your partner use his thumbs and three fingers, pressing hard for from three to seven seconds.

4. Now find the points on your upper back between and above your shoulder blades. This is your interscapular area. Have your partner apply pressure for from three to seven seconds.

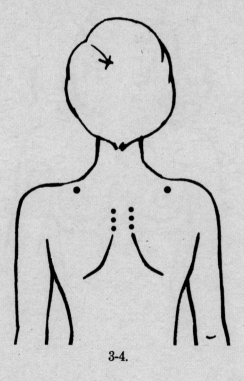

3-4.

5. Place your hands on your breasts in an open position. The best position for this treatment is lying down. Knead your breasts, using an outward, circular movement. This should be done for from three to seven seconds.

5.

Chapter Six

CHILDREN CAN BENEFIT, TOO

Acupressure, as a part of your child's regular care, can be a relaxing, pleasuring, healthful and beneficial form of contact between mother or father and baby.

As with your own acupressure self-treatment, your baby's care can take place during the normal daily routine—before and after the bath, during diapering, or before bedtime.

Parents who have tried acupressure report that their children have improved appetites, healthier bowel action, and increased rates of growth. They also feel that they have more relaxed, happier babies.

Here's something you can do while diapering your baby:

1. Locate points near your baby's navel. Press lightly, then gradually increase pressure for from three to seven seconds.

2. Now, apply pressure to the pit of the stomach with the balls of your fingers. Apply pressure for two seconds.

3. The next area to treat is the area below the navel and over the bladder. Using three fingers, gently press three times.

4. Use your palms to press the navel five times.

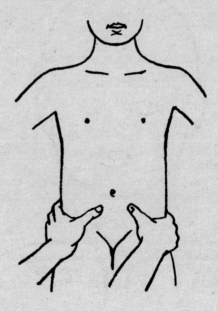

WRYNECK IN CHILDREN

Some children develop a condition of the neck called wryneck. The neck muscles become shortened, hardened and contracted. This condition is congenital in some children; in others it is caused by sleeping predominantly on one side. Of course, if your child's condition is severe, see a doctor.

You can treat your child's sterno-mastoid muscle and avoid the mild form of this condition.

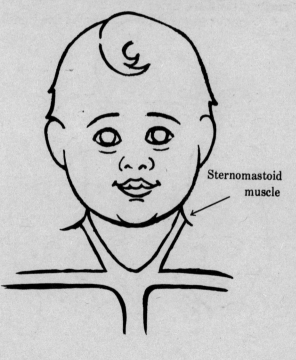

Sternomastoid muscle

1. Locate the hardened, contracted muscles in the neck. You may use your thumbs to work downward, and apply pressure in these areas.

2. Locate the points in the front of the neck. Then travel in a line from below the ear to the tip of the shoulder. Apply pressure for from three to seven seconds. Repeat ten times.

3. Locate the points at the side of the neck. Press for three to seven seconds. Do this ten times. Take care to be gentle. Be thorough and consistent, however.

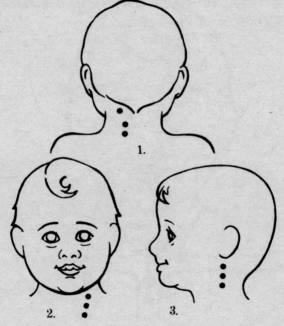

BEDWETTING

Bedwetting problems are common in children. Sometimes it is because they worry, or sometimes they are tense. Sometimes the reaction of the sphincter in the bladder is dulled. They may become chilled during sleep. They may have taken too much liquid during the day. No matter what the cause, here are some treatments that should bring an end to your child's bedwetting problems.

1. Locate the points on the lumbar region and the three points on the sacrum. Press for from three to seven seconds.

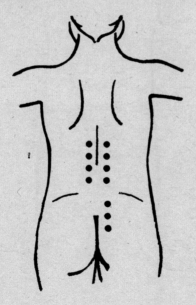

2. Locate the points on the lower abdomen, especially those over the bladder. Press with the palm of the hand for from three to seven seconds.

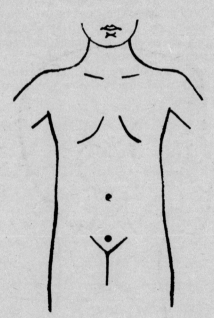

3. Locate the point over the medulla oblongata, or low brain. It is at the upper part of the back of the neck. Press gently with the thumbs for from three to seven seconds.

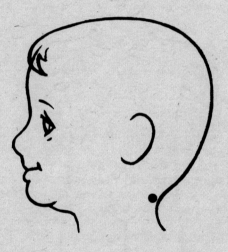

Chapter Seven

MORE ABOUT ACUPRESSURE

In this book, I have presented material that the reader can use in the self-treatment of the ordinary aches and pains of everyday life.

In the following pages, I will attempt to give some background on acupressure and answer some questions that may have been raised.

A Word About Meridian Therapy

Acupressure is a major form of meridian therapy, that is, a treatment of energy points based on the theory that lines or meridians of energy are constantly flowing (in a constant direction) through the body in set patterns, much as the nervous system sends impulses or as the circulatory system sends blood to all organs and extremities of the body.

Acupressure is based on the premise that when a person's *chi*, or life energy, is in balance, the body works in a more efficient way, with stress equally distributed throughout the system, thus maintaining a high level of resistance to disease and toxins.

Certain tonification points are used routinely on a periodic basis in order to help insure the normal, healthy flow of energy. Tonification is an increase of energy concentration, or excitation of energy, in a meridian (sometimes to affect a particular organ or area of the body).

When the free flow of energy is interrupted, or when one part of the body becomes overactive (or underactive) because of improper diet, lack of rest or exercise, or too much stress, treatment of various tonification points may help to stimulate or sedate a meridian (or portion of a meridian) in order to help bring the energy flow back into balance once again.

About the Meridians

The body is divided into twelve major meridians or channels, according to meridian therapy. Each meridian has a right and left half. The energy, however, flows continuously and unbroken through the body—or it should.

Each part of the body and each function is controlled by at least one of these major meridians. Ten of the meridians are named for the organs and functions with which they are related: These are the spleen, the stomach, the lung, the large intestine, the kidney, the bladder, the liver, the gallbladder, the heart, and the small intestine.

The other two major meridians, the triple-warmer, or tri-heater and the circulation-sex or heart constrictor are more related to functions than to specific organs.

The tri-heater is associated with the use and transfer of energy, including the exchange of gasses in the lungs, use of energy in the digestive process and in the genital-urinary functions.

The heart-constrictor is literally translated as "envelope of the heart." Its function is to give protection to the heart and to control heart action and other functions, including circulation and reproduction.

The Midline Meridians

Besides the twelve major meridians, there are two vertical meridians that encircle the midline of the body in front and back.

The conception vessel (or vessel of conception) extends up the front of the body from the center of the perineum to the lower lip. The governing vessel extends up the length of the back of the body from the coccyx up to and over the head down the face to the upper lip.

The function of these unilateral meridians is to store and unite to *Chi*, the energy or life force, thus helping all other meridians work together.

The governing vessel acts for *yang* meridian activity, and the conception vessel for *yin* meridian activity. (See section on *yin* and *yang*.)

On the following pages, I will list the major meridians and their paths through the body.

The Paths of the Major Meridians

1. *Spleen:* Begins at the top outside tip of the big toe, goes up inside of the leg, up the torso to the front of the shoulder, then halfway down the sides of the chest.
2. *Stomach:* This meridian goes in two lines, from eye to chin and side of the head to the chin. It connects with and goes down the neck, torso, and front of the leg, to the outside of the toe.
3. *Lung:* This meridian begins just in front of the shoulder. It extends down the inside of the arm to the inside of the thumb.
4. *Large Intestine:* The large intestine meridian begins at the tip of the first finger and extends up and outside of the arm, over the shoulder to the front of the neck up the face to the side of the nose.
5. *Kidney:* The kidney meridian begins on the bottom of the foot. It goes up the back and inside of the leg between the thighs up the front of the torso to the top of the sternum.
6. *Bladder:* The bladder meridian begins between the eyes, at the top of the nose. It extends over the head, down the back (up and down in two lines). It goes down the back of the leg to the calf.
7. *Liver:* The liver meridian begins between the big toe and the second toe. It goes up the inside of the leg, and continues up the thigh to the pubic area.
8. *Gallbladder:* The gallbladder meridian begins at the outside corner of the eye. It zigzags back

and forth in curves on the side of the head, around the back of the shoulders, to the front of the chest and down the outside of the body and leg to the tip of the fourth toe.

9. *Heart:* This meridian goes from the armpit down inside of the arm to the palm. It ends just below the little finger.

10. *Small Intestine:* The small intestine meridian goes from the tip of the little finger on the top of the hand up the arm to the back of the shoulder, up the side of the neck, to the cheek, to the front of the ear.

11. *Tri-Heater:* The tri-heater or triple warmer meridian runs from the top tip of the fourth finger, up the arm over the shoulder to the base of the skull. It runs over the ear to the eye.

12. *Heart Constrictor:* The heart constrictor meridian begins at the base of the fingers near the center of the palm. It goes up the arm and ends at the chest.

13. *Conception Vessel:* The conception vessel meridian extends up the front of the body from the perineum to the lower lip.

14. *Governing Vessel:* The governing vessel meridian extends up the length of the back from the coccyx up to and over the head down the face to the upper lip.

Energy in Acupressure

I have said that acupressure is involved with balancing the body's energy. To understand this better, we must understand how the Orientals envision the concept of energy.

The Chi: In traditional Chinese and Japanese philosophy, it is believed there is a motivating force behind all life, called *chi.*

This life force or vital energy, basic to all meridian therapy in theory and practice, controls the balance or harmony and wellbeing of the body and mind. The *chi* is also said to be the manifestation of the Tao (the basic creative principle of the entire universe as conceived by Taoists) in the body. It is considered the life-force energy.

The *chi* is believed to flow through the twelve major meridians in a constant pulsing daily pattern of circulation. In fact, there is a biological clock; each meridian has a two-hour peak period each day.

The Yin and Yang: The *chi* consists of two aspects, the *yin* (negative) and the *yang* (positive). These influences act as delicate pulses throughout the body. They undulate similar to the tides, and it is the balance between these influences that is necessary to maintain harmony or health in the body.

Yin and *yang* are contained within each other; they are defined as existing only together, in much the same way as night and day.

The qualities of *yin* are considered negative: dark, moon, winter, receptivity. The meridians with paths along the inside of the body, e.g. under the arm, are called the *yin* meridians.

The qualities of *yang* are light, sunny, summer, aggressive, reaching out. The meridians with paths that move along the outside or sunny side of the body are called the *yang* meridians.

The Five-Element Theory: Chi, as it operates in the body, is further divided in the interrelationship of forces. The Chinese originally explained these aspects or stages of *chi* in parables or stories most people could easily understand.

Thus, these five aspects (each containing *yin* and *yang* forces) are called wood, fire, earth, metal and water.

In terms of acupressure, and meridian therapy, certain meridians are related to each of these elements. Therefore, the system is a basis for determining treatment of a particular meridian, as it relates to organs of the body.

To give an example of how the parable works: There are two cycles, the *Shin,* or engendering cycle and the *K'O* or controlling cycle.

The *Shin,* or engendering cycle is explained this way: Earth gives birth to metal, which "grows" in the earth; water condenses around metal, and is thus "formed" from metal, water makes the growth of wood (plants, life) possible; wood is the fuel of fire; fire leaves ashes as remains that become earth again.

The *K'O,* or controlling cycle is explained this way: The earth dams water; water puts out fire; fire melts metal; metal cuts wood; and wood digs earth.

The Master

A master of meridian therapy is usually a highly skilled, well-educated, experienced, practitioner of this very involved healing art. He is sometimes referred to as a Doctor of Acupuncture. His education involves both theory and practice.

True masters from the Orient have usually undergone intensive training and formal teaching by instructors and medical examiners.

In the past, a master's reputation rested on his ability to keep his patients healthy. For this he was paid regularly. When his patients became ill, his fees stopped until they regained their health.

In the United States, acupressure practitioners usually find a master to study with and accept his verdict as to when they are ready to practice on their own.

You may find a master by contacting the acupuncture and acupressure research projects associated with the major hospitals. Today there are many medical doctors who are becoming familiar with acupressure and may be able to refer you to a reputable master.

FIVE ELEMENTS CHART

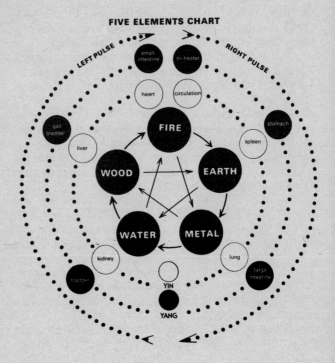

CONCLUSION

In the 1960s, people in the United States began to be more aware of the interrelationships between mind and body. Yoga regained popularity, the Oriental martial arts, such as Judo, Jujitsu, Kung Fu, Aikido, came to enjoy a large following of enthusiastic students. Western forms of body/mind therapy, such as bioenergetics, Reichian and neo-Reichian work and the Feldenkreis method, became popular.

Along with all of this, there came an increasing awareness of the importance of touch to an individual's well-being. We discovered that the body/mind split was placing Western man and woman under ever-increasing stress.

Beginning with Yoga and the martial arts, Americans started to search out the literature of various Eastern philosophers and to learn all they could from them. Words like *chi, yin* and *yang* began to crop up in everyday conversations.

Massage, nude encounter, ways of getting the body in on the human potential act blossomed toward the end of the sixties and into the seventies. Also, stress began to be studied scientifically. A third factor, an interest in natural foods and self-healing, combined to make acupressure a natural concern for people already interested in getting as much as they can out of life.

In addition to being a popular new form of massage therapy, acupressure, proven valuable throughout the ages, is now considered an effective healing device and preventive health measure.

APPENDIX

ACUPRESSURE IN TREATMENT OF SERIOUS DISORDERS

Acupressure treatment of serious diseases demands the careful attention of a master. You should not attempt to treat yourself, and you should have a check-up by a physician before you subject yourself to acupressure for any physical problem.

I include these treatments to illustrate the great possibilities of acupressure in dealing with serious illnesses.

GASTRALGIA

Sudden and acute pains on the right side, or in the pit of the stomach, may mean gastralgia, a disorder of the gallbladder.

To treat gastralgia, a master will have you rest on your stomach, then he will straddle your body and place his right thumb on a point between your shoulder blades.

He will put his left thumb on top of the right one, and press with the full weight of his body for five seconds. He will repeat this five or six times.

If you still complain of pain, he will apply pressure along the sides of your vertebrae.

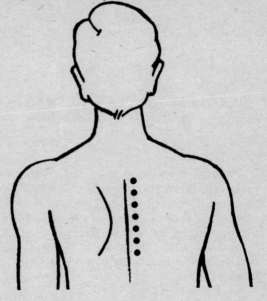

He will then have you turn over on your back, and press the pit of your stomach lightly with the palm of his hand.

COMMON COLD

To clear up nasal congestion, the master will:
1. Press firmly on the front of the neck.
2. Next, using the middle finger placed on top of the index finger, apply repeated pressure to both sides of the nose, from the root to the nostrils. This should clear up the congestion.

HOARSENESS

1. Press repeatedly on the third and fourth points in the front of the neck.
2. Apply gentle finger pressure to the occipital region, the upper shoulder, and the solar plexus (pit of the stomach).

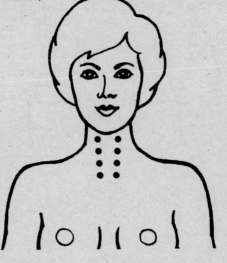

RHEUMATISM

Here's what an acupressure master might do if you came to him for rheumatism treatments:

1. Have you sit upright, and kneel beside him with one knee drawn up.

2. He would then apply pressure, first to the key points of the deltoid muscle in the shoulder, and then work downward. He might repeat this three times for two seconds each. Once he reaches the area of greatest pain, it is likely that you will react, showing him the root of the problem.

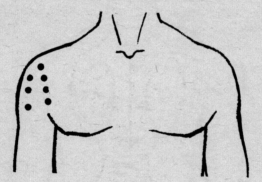

3. Here's another treatment: You recline on your side with your back to the doctor. With one thumb after the other he will apply pressure to the three points below the hollow of the scapula. Since the area will be very sensitive, he will begin with light pressure and gradually increase the force.

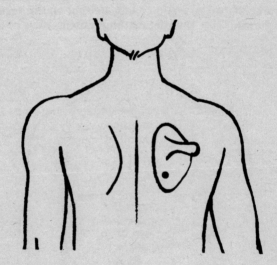

Another acupressure treatment for rheumatism is centered on the back:

1. The master will have you recline face down; he will sit beside you.

2. Using three fingers, he will press the fifth lumbar vertebra lightly. You will feel pain at the point requiring treatment.

3. The master will then apply pressure simultaneously with both thumbs to the muscles on either side of the vertebra, but not on the vertebra itself. After the surrounding muscles have relaxed, he will press the vertebra. He will continue the pressure until you report some easing of the condition.

4. Then he will have you lie on your back.

5. Sitting beside you, he will press lightly with the palm of his hand on your abdomen. Once he finds the hard area, he will press until you relax that muscle. When your abdomen relaxes, the pain in your lower back should disappear.

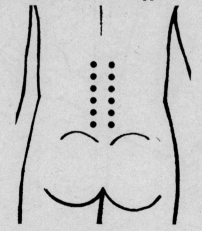

NOSEBLEED

Here's what an acupressure master might do for you if you come to him with chronic nosebleeding:

Holding your forehead with his left hand, he might massage the points on the medulla oblongata with his right thumb till the bleeding stops.

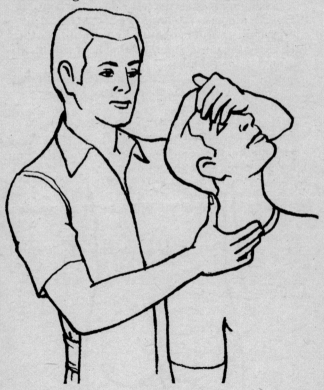

SLIPPED DISC (spinal)

Here what a master might do for you if you had a slipped disk:

1. First he would ask you where the pain is. He would determine whether it is on the right or left side of the body.

2. Assuming it is on the left side of the body, at the fourth lumbar vertebra, here is the treatment:

3. Avoiding abrupt pressure, he would relieve the stiffness of the muscle on the left side by continual pressure of the thumbs.

4. Next, he would use the bulb of the middle finger to softly press the concave spot between the fourth and fifth vertebrae.

5. He would press lightly for a duration of one second, then repeat five times.

6. He might have you turn over on your back, and apply pressure with the fingers and the palm to your abdominal region, paying close attention to the pit of the stomach.

7. The next step is the pressure on the points around the navel.

8. Finally, he will apply palm pressure to any area in the lumbar region where you complain of pain.

9. Some masters require that you rest for a few days after this treatment.

WHIPLASH

Here's the finger pressure treatment for whiplash:
Locate the points at the sides and back of the neck, and the area from the base of the medulla oblongata to the base of the neck. Press for five to seven seconds. This should return the muscles in the back of the neck, and also the slipped bones, to their normal positions.

Many masters recommend an immediate application of acupressure after any injury, as these distortions do not always show up in an X ray.

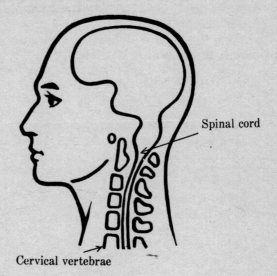

Spinal cord

Cervical vertebrae

Here's how a master might treat your motion sickness!

First he presses the point at the base of the kneecap, the *sanri*. Then he might treat the plantar arches, the medulla oblongata, and the nape of the neck.

For airsickness, pressure on the mastoid bone, the temples, the medulla oblongata, and the nape of the neck is often considered the best treatment.

For seasickness, you should remain quiet. Then apply pressure to the mastoid region, the abdomen (especially the gastric region), the upper shoulder, and the backbone.

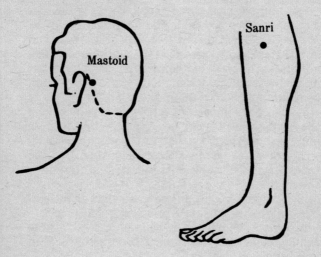

LACK OF FEELING IN THE LEGS

Some people complain about an absence of feeling, or numbness in the legs after sitting or standing too long. Here's what a master might do for you if have this problem:

1. Apply pressure to the eight points on the calf muscle.
2. Lightly massage the six points on the ankle with both hands.
3. Press the point in front of the knee, the *sanri*.
4. Press the ankle.
5. Press the sole of the foot.

TOOTHACHE DUE TO TENSION

For any toothache, you should see your dentist. Yet some aches are as much due to tension in the jaw, as to actual difficulties with your teeth and gums. Here's a treatment that could be a welcome adjunct to the care your dentist gives you. It is what an acupressure master might do, if you went to him complaining about a toothache:

1. There are important acupressure points along the carotid artery under the lower jaw. Locate these and press on the same side as the aching tooth.
2. Press the points along the temple. Use the three fingers. This will be repeated two or three times.
3. Locate the point on the lower part of the ear. Press along the jaw until you reach that point.
4. Locate the part of the cheek directly over the aching tooth. Press for three to seven seconds. Pain will begin to subside.

HEADACHE

Here's what a master might do for you if you have
been unsuccessful in treating your own headaches.
Remember, headaches can be a symptom of severe
organic diseases. First, see your doctor for persist-
ent headaches. If your doctor finds nothing wrong, a
master might try the following:

1. Locate the points of the median line, from the
hairline to the crown of your head.

2. Apply pressure to the key points on the left
and right of the crown.

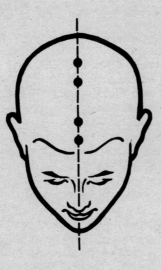

INDEX